Natural Heartburn Relief

A Beginner's 2-Week Step-by-Step Guide With Sample Curated Recipes and a Sample Meal Plan

mf

copyright © 2024 Tyler Spellmann

All rights reserved No part of this book may be reproduced, or stored in a retrieval system, or transmitted in any form or by any means, electronic, mechanical, photocopying, recording, or otherwise, without express written permission of the publisher.

Disclaimer

By reading this disclaimer, you are accepting the terms of the disclaimer in full. If you disagree with this disclaimer, please do not read the guide.

All of the content within this guide is provided for informational and educational purposes only, and should not be accepted as independent medical or other professional advice. The author is not a doctor, physician, nurse, mental health provider, or registered nutritionist/dietician. Therefore, using and reading this guide does not establish any form of a physician-patient relationship.

Always consult with a physician or another qualified health provider with any issues or questions you might have regarding any sort of medical condition. Do not ever disregard any qualified professional medical advice or delay seeking that advice because of anything you have read in this guide. The information in this guide is not intended to be any sort of medical advice and should not be used in lieu of any medical advice by a licensed and qualified medical professional.

The information in this guide has been compiled from a variety of known sources. However, the author cannot attest to or guarantee the accuracy of each source and thus should not be held liable for any errors or omissions.

You acknowledge that the publisher of this guide will not be held liable for any loss or damage of any kind incurred as a result of this guide or the reliance on any information provided within this guide. You acknowledge and agree that you assume all risk and responsibility for any action you undertake in response to the information in this guide.

Using this guide does not guarantee any particular result (e.g., weight loss or a cure). By reading this guide, you acknowledge that there are no guarantees to any specific outcome or results you can expect.

All product names, diet plans, or names used in this guide are for identification purposes only and are the property of their respective owners. The use of these names does not imply endorsement. All other trademarks cited herein are the property of their respective owners.

Where applicable, this guide is not intended to be a substitute for the original work of this diet plan and is, at most, a supplement to the original work for this diet plan and never a direct substitute. This guide is a personal expression of the facts of that diet plan.

Where applicable, persons shown in the cover images are stock photography models and the publisher has obtained the rights to use the images through license agreements with third-party stock image companies.

Table of Contents

Introduction	**8**
Getting to Know Heartburn	**10**
What is heartburn?	10
What are its symptoms?	10
Countering Heartburn	**13**
Foods That Are Good and Bad for Heartburn	**16**
Foods that trigger acid reflux are the following:	17
Commonly bad foods for reflux	18
Foods okay for reflux	19
Creating Your Heartburn Diary	**23**
The 7-Day Diet Plan	**26**
Sunday	26
Monday	26
Tuesday	27
Wednesday	27
Thursday	27
Friday	28
Saturday	28
Heartburn Relief Recipes	**29**
Banana Ginger Smoothie	30
Gala Apple Honeydew Smoothie	31
Muesli-Style Oatmeal	32
Instant Polenta with Sesame Seeds	33
Calm Carrot Salad	34
Black Bean and Cilantro Soup	35
Flavorful Cantaloupe Gazpacho	36
Creamy Hummus	37
Watermelon and Ginger Granite	38
Quick Banana Sorbet	39
Marinated Tuna Steak	40

Honey Roasted Potatoes	41
Kale Banana Smoothie	42
Maple Salmon	43
Vegetable Broth	44
Spinach and Chickpeas	46
Apple Cinnamon Smash Oatmeal	47
Fruit and Dark Greens Salad	48
Spinach, Feta, and Tomato Omelet	50
Salmon and Asparagus	51
Grilled Eggplant	52
Physical Activity and Heartburn Management	**53**
Understanding the Connection	53
Choosing the Right Exercise	54
Hydration and Heartburn	54
Heartburn-Friendly Workout Plan	55
Other Lifestyle Remedies to Manage Heartburn	**56**
Stress Management	56
Weight Management	56
Smoking and Alcohol	57
Clothing Choices	57
Proper Posture	57
Adequate Sleep	57
Medication Review	58
A Two-Week Guide to Managing Heartburn	**59**
Day 1-3: Dietary Changes	59
Day 4-5: Meal Planning	59
Day 6-7: Exercise Incorporation	59
Day 8-10: Wardrobe Adjustment	60
Day 11-12: Posture and Sleep Adjustment	60
Day 13-14: Medication Review	60
Conclusion	**61**

Introduction

Heartburn is a common problem for millions of people around the world. Experts say, there are about 15 million Americans who are experiencing heartburn each day based on research conducted by the American College of Gastroenterology.

The goal of this guide is to help you with the following:

- Understanding what heartburn is and differentiating it from other conditions
- Learning about different ways to control and counter heartburn with food
- Planning a two-week heartburn relief diet plan
- Introducing different recipes to support the heartburn relief diet

Before proceeding into the two-week heartburn relief diet plan, make sure that you are committed to this by being disciplined and determined. It's important to start this diet with the mindset because you might need to change or stop some habits in order to make your diet plan a successful one.

Take drinking too much coffee for example. When you are in the process of lowering your stomach acidity, you need to avoid or lessen your intake of acidic foods and beverages like coffee. We all know that coffee is an addictive drink because it contains caffeine. As much as it is addictive, it is also very high in acid.

Caffeine withdrawal is hard and can result in some adverse effects for people who drink it several times a day. The bad effects can be headaches, fatigue, anxiety, difficulty in concentrating, irritability, tremors, and low energy levels. If you are a certified coffee addict, you might experience these side effects.

The point is, that you might be obliged to do new things and leave your old habits during and after accomplishing the diet plan. The challenge here is to impose discipline on yourself.

If you're ready to start this journey and are willing to take on the challenge, go ahead and proceed in reading this guide.

Getting to Know Heartburn

What is heartburn?

Heartburn is an acid reflux symptom where you can feel a burning sensation in your lower chest, specifically behind your breastbone. This happens when the contents of the stomach go back up to the esophagus. Commonly, the symptoms worsen after eating big portions of meals or when you lay down.

What are its symptoms?

Usually, when you experience a heartburn, you feel like your chest is burning. However, some chest pains can be signs of another medical condition. It is best to talk to your doctor personally for proper medication. Here are some symptoms that can help you determine if that feeling of your chest burning is heartburn:

- Burning sensations in your chest, particularly behind your breastbone, can last for a few minutes up to some hours.

- You feel the pain in your chest every time you bend over or lay down.
- You also feel burning sensations in your throat.
- There can be a sour, hot, salty, or acidic taste in your throat.
- You cannot swallow easily.
- You feel nauseous.

How is it different from GERD and acid reflux?

Most people think heartburn, GERD, and acid reflux are all the same. This is a common misconception, which is not entirely wrong because these three are somewhat related as well.

According to the Gastroenterologist of Cleveland Clinic, Scott Gabbard, MD, acid reflux is described as a type of disorder where the valve that separates the stomach and esophagus opens at times when it is not supposed to open. As an effect, the stomach contents such as the digestive juices, acids, and food from the stomach go back up to the esophagus.

He added that there are times when people don't immediately feel refluxes even when they're already having it for almost an hour.

Meanwhile, GERD, or Gastroesophageal reflux disease is a higher form of acid reflux. It is more severe than acid reflux.

Gastroesophageal reflux disease or GERD requires treatment to prevent more serious health problems in the long run.

How come some over-the-counter medicines don't work with acid reflux?

The reason for heartburn caused by acid reflux can be a little complicated. Experts say that it is not actually because of stomach acid. It is because of pepsin. Pepsin is a digestive enzyme that breaks down protein and can only perform its job when acids are present. In other words, it is the pepsin molecules that eat digestive linings and not the acid. The acid here serves as the fuel for pepsin molecules to activate. Thus, there might be instances when medicines cannot alleviate the symptoms.

Countering Heartburn

There are ways to counter heartburn. Here are some tips that will help you alleviate the symptoms as soon as you start to feel that you're experiencing heartburn:

Stand up. This can ease the sensation you are feeling. In case this doesn't work out, correct your posture as you stand up. This might help.

In case you're lying down, prop up your upper body with pillows. Laying down without elevating your upper body can worsen the burning sensation.

Wear loose clothes. This helps minimize the discomfort you are feeling brought by the burning sensation in your chest. For women, do not wear bras.

Try drinking baking soda and water mixture. Baking soda is known for its ability to neutralize stomach acid. Baking soda or sodium bicarbonate is a base and has a pH level of around 8 to 9.

Drink teas that are good for alleviating heartburns like chamomile tea. Be careful of choosing the tea you will drink because most types of tea can trigger heartburn.

Put grated ginger roots in your teas or soup. In Chinese medicine, ginger is used to cure ailments. It can help you to relieve nausea. Ginger is also known to help in reducing the likelihood of stomach acid to back up the esophagus. However, take note that this has to be taken in small doses because large doses of ginger can trigger additional heartburn instead.

Other than these tips, there are also lifestyle changes that can help prevent heartburn from occurring in the first place. These include:

- Avoid foods and drinks that can trigger heartburn such as spicy, fatty, or acidic foods.
- Eat smaller meals more frequently instead of large meals to avoid putting too much pressure on the stomach.
- Chew gum after meals to increase saliva production which can help neutralize stomach acid.
- Sip on water throughout the day to dilute stomach acid and maintain proper hydration.
- Avoid lying down immediately after eating, as this can cause stomach acid to flow back up into the esophagus.

- Maintain a healthy weight to reduce pressure on the stomach and prevent heartburn.

There are also over-the-counter medications available to help alleviate heartburn symptoms. Antacids like Tums or Rolaids can provide quick relief by neutralizing stomach acid. H2 blockers, such as Pepcid and Zantac, decrease the production of stomach acid. Proton pump inhibitors (PPIs) like Prilosec and Nexium block acid production in the stomach for longer-lasting relief. However, it is important to consult with a doctor before taking any medication, as they may have potential side effects or interact with other medications.

Foods That Are Good and Bad for Heartburn

Some people who suffer from acid reflux and go to a medical expert are prescribed over-the-counter medications, such as a histamine-2 blocker in particular. These OTC medicines like Tagamet cimetidine, famotidine, or ranitidine are known to subdue the secretion of stomach acids and can alleviate symptoms of acid reflux.

For people experiencing a more severe condition, proton pump inhibitors are commonly prescribed to them. Examples of these are lansoprazole, pantoprazole, and omeprazole. Proton pump inhibitors almost stop all stomach acid secretions.

Meanwhile, there are those who don't respond to these kinds of medications and are advised to undergo minimally invasive surgeries.

If you want to prevent problematic acid refluxes that will cause you pains in the chest while also avoiding the need to take medications, you need to be mindful of what you have to change in your diet. Below is a great list to start with.

Foods that trigger acid reflux are the following:

Food with high acid content:
- Sodas and all carbonated juices or drinks
- Alcoholic drinks
- Vinegar
- Fruits that belong to the citrus family like lemons, limes, grapefruits, and oranges

Food with high-fat content:
- Fatty meats like sausages, ribs, and bacon
- Deep-fried foods
- Nuts
- Cream sauce
- Margarine, butter, shortening, and lard
- Chocolates
- Drinks that are high in caffeine like coffee and tea
- Mints like spearmint and peppermint
- Hot sauces
- Pepper

Commonly bad foods for reflux

Acidic foods

- Tomatoes, tomato juice, tomato sauce, tomato paste
- Apples and applesauce
- Onions
- Cucumber
- Garlic
- Green peppers
- Nuts
- Some herbal teas, with the exception of chamomile tea
- Spicy foods

Other acidic foods

- Sauces and condiments
- Barbecue sauce
- Hot sauce
- Caesar dressing
- Mustard
- Ketchup
- Ranch dressing
- Pickles
- Salsa
- Worcestershire sauce
- Russian dressing
- Thousand Island dressing
- Fruits

- Grapes
- Blackberries
- Peaches
- Cherries
- Strawberries
- Blueberries
- Cranberries, cranberry juice
- Mango
- Kiwi
- Pomegranate
- Pineapple
- Full-fat milk
- Iced tea
- V8 vegetable juice
- Full-fat yogurt

Foods okay for reflux

Now that we've identified foods that can trigger acid reflux, let's focus on foods that can manage the acid levels in your stomach. These foods are what you must have in your two-week diet plan to minimize acid refluxes as they are strictly non-acidic foods. Here are the list of foods to follow during the two-week induction phase:

Proteins

- Skinless chicken – broiled, grilled, steamed, or baked
- Organic fish and poultry

- Tofu
- Egg whites
- Turkey breast, organic and skinless
- Fish, including shellfish – sushi, broiled, grilled, steamed, or baked

Carbs

- Bagels
- Pasta, with non-acidic sauce
- Beans
- Bread – unprocessed wheat, rye, whole grain
- Muffins – low-fat and non-fruit
- Whole-grain cereals and oatmeal
- Popcorn – no butter, plain or salted
- Rice
- Breakfast cereals, crackers

Fruits with low acid content

- Pears, preferably ripe, 4 pcs. per week
- Bananas
- Red apples
- Melons – honeydew, watermelon, cantaloupe

Vegetables that have low acid content

- Fennel
- Green vegetables, except bell pepper
- Parsley

- Mushrooms, cooked or raw
- Potatoes
- Turnips
- Vegetables, cooked or raw, except for tomato
- Root vegetables, all but raw onions
- Red bell peppers, maximum of one per week

Condiments and dressings

- Vinaigrette – 1 tbsp. a day
- Honey mustard
- Low-fat dressings

Sweeteners

- Honey
- Agave nectar
- Caramel, maximum of 4 tbsp. a week
- Non-natural sweetener, maximum of 2 tsp. a day

Beverages

- Non-carbonated water
- Coffee, preferably with milk, 1 cup a day
- Chamomile tea

Others

- Bouillon or chicken stock
- Aloe vera
- Olive oil, 1 to 2 tbsp. a day

- Ginger, preserved or powdered, or ginger root
- Milk or soy milk – fat-free, 2 percent, or free from lactose
- Herbs, except for peppers, mustard, and citrus
- Homemade soups, preferably with low-acid veggies and noodles

Creating Your Heartburn Diary

Now let's go to the very essence of this heartburn relief diet guide. The goal here is to give your esophagus, throat membrane linings, and other parts of the digestive tract that are affected by acid reflux, the chance to heal.

The two-week relief diet program can be summarized as maintaining a low-acid and low-fat diet and refraining yourself from foods that may trigger acid reflux. For example, fruits are generally prohibited, but bananas and melons are okay. For your liquid intake, water will be your main beverage. Make sure you consume at least 8 glasses of water a day.

To help you track what you eat and which ones worsen your heartburn, creating a daily food diary is highly encouraged. A food diary will help your doctor properly diagnose your symptoms by looking at the list of foods that affect your heartburn.

You'll keep a record of your diet during this two-week diet plan. In your diary, write how often you feel the burning sensation. Take note of the time when the symptoms occur—in some instances, you might have to record more than one occurrence. Make sure that your records are free from any errors.

To start making your diary, create five columns. Each column will be captioned: time, food/drink, amount (of food or drinks you are taking for that particular time), activity, and the symptoms that occurred after. Here is an example of the diary:

Time	Food/Drink	Amount	Activity	Symptoms
6:00 am	Bread toast	2 slices	At home having a wonderful breakfast	None
	Boiled egg	1 pc.	in the kitchen.	
	Melon juice	medium, 4 oz.		
7:00 am	Coffee with creamer	12 oz.	Reading the daily news	Sour taste
10:45 am	Banana	1 pc., large	Watching TV shows	None
12:30 pm	Rice	1 cup	Just having lunch	None
	Fish soup	1 small bowl		

3:00 pm	Coffee with milk	12 oz.	Attending a ZOOM meeting	Sour taste
6:00 pm	Grilled chicken (without skin)	small portion	Dinner	None
7:00 pm	Chamomile tea	1 small cup	Relaxing	None

Note that this is only a sample diary. You can have your way of recording your daily activities, just be accurate when jotting them down. Then, share this information with our doctor for a more accurate diagnosis.

The 7-Day Diet Plan

Now, let's get into our two-week heartburn relief diet plan. Here's a detailed seven days meal plan for you:

Sunday

Breakfast: Apple Cinnamon Smash Oatmeal

Morning snacks: Banana Ginger Smoothie

Lunch: Vegetable Broth

Afternoon snacks: Creamy Hummus

Dinner: Chicken Salad

Monday

Breakfast: Spinach, Feta, and Tomato Omelet

Morning snacks: Gala Apple Honeydew Smoothie

Lunch: Orange-Walnut Salad

Afternoon snacks: Banana Ginger Smoothie

Dinner: Maple Salmon

Tuesday

Breakfast: Muesli-Style Oatmeal

Morning snacks: Ripe bananas

Lunch: Calm Carrot Salad

Afternoon snacks: Kale Banana Smoothie

Dinner: Spinach and Watercress Salad

Wednesday

Breakfast: Instant Polenta with Sesame Seeds

Morning snacks: Creamy Hummus

Lunch: **Spinach** and Chickpeas

Afternoon snacks: Watermelon and Ginger Granite

Dinner: Grilled Eggplant with Plain Rice

Thursday

Breakfast: Honey Roasted Potatoes

Morning snacks: Gala Apple Honeydew Smoothie

Lunch: Apple Cinnamon Smash Oatmeal

Afternoon snacks: Quick Banana Sorbet

Dinner: Maple Salmon

Friday

Breakfast: Apple Cinnamon Smash Oatmeal

Morning snacks: Kale Banana Smoothie

Lunch: Zucchini, Celery Greens Soup

Afternoon snacks: Quick Banana Sorbet

Dinner: Black Bean and Cilantro Soup

Saturday

Breakfast: Muesli-Style Oatmeal

Morning snacks: Creamy Hummus

Lunch: Grilled Eggplant with Plain Rice

Afternoon snacks: Flavorful Cantaloupe Gazpacho

Dinner: Marinated Tuna Steak

Heartburn Relief Recipes

Banana Ginger Smoothie

Ingredients:

- 2 pcs. ripe bananas
- 2 cups milk
- 1 cup yogurt
- ½ cup ice
- ½ tsp. garlic, peeled and shredded
- Optional: 2 tbsp. honey or brown sugar

Instructions:

1. Blend all the ingredients until smooth.
2. Serve.

Gala Apple Honeydew Smoothie

Ingredients:

- 1 pc. Gala apple
- 2 cups Honeydew melon
- 4 tbsp. fresh aloe vera, peeled
- 1 ½ cups ice
- 1/16 tsp. lime zest
- ¼ tsp. salt

Instructions:

1. Peel, deseed, and slice the apple and honeydew melon. Don't forget to follow the suggested quantity above.
2. Put them in a blender together with the peeled fresh aloe vera, ice, lime zest, and salt.
3. Blend until smooth. Start from low to high blending. After that, stir.

Muesli-Style Oatmeal

Ingredients:

- ½ banana, diced
- 1 cup instant oatmeal
- 1/2 golden apple, peeled and diced
- 1 cup milk
- 2 tbsp. raisins
- 2 tsp. honey or sugar
- A pinch of salt

Instructions:

1. In a bowl, mix oatmeal, raisins, milk, sugar or honey, and salt.
2. Put a cover and refrigerate.
3. Leave the mixture overnight for at least 2 hours.
4. Get it out of the fridge after the allotted time then serve with fruits.
5. Add some milk if the mixture gets too thick.

Instant Polenta with Sesame Seeds

Ingredients:

- ¾ cup instant polenta or cornmeal
- 3 tbsp. brown sugar
- 3 cups whole milk
- 1 tbsp. sesame seeds
- ½ tsp. vanilla extract
- 1 tsp. orange extract
- Salt, to taste

Instructions:

1. Boil milk.
2. Add instant polenta or cornmeal. Stir to avoid lumps until cooked.
3. When cooked, add orange extract, vanilla, brown sugar, and salt.
4. Add the sesame seeds to the top upon serving.

Calm Carrot Salad

Ingredients:

- 1 lb. grated carrots
- 2 tbsp. raisins
- ¼ lb. mesclun greens
- 1 tsp. dried oregano
- 2 tbsp. orange juice
- 2 tbsp. brown sugar
- ¼ tsp. salt
- 2 tsp. olive oil

Instructions:

1. For the dressing, mix orange juice, raisins, brown sugar, oregano, salt, and olive oil in a bowl. Leave it for five minutes.
2. Mix the dressing and carrots thoroughly.
3. Add salt if necessary.
4. Put it over the mesclun leaves then serve.

Black Bean and Cilantro Soup

Ingredients:

- 8 oz. canned black beans
- 1/2 cup cilantro
- 1 pint chicken stock
- 1 tbsp. sour cream, nonfat
- Salt, to taste

Instructions:

1. Boil chicken stock.
2. Put the cilantro and beans.
3. Season with salt.
4. Cook in low heat for 30 minutes.
5. Blend until the desired texture is achieved.
6. Add some salt if needed.
7. Put it in a bowl then top it with sour cream and cilantro.
8. Serve and enjoy.

Flavorful Cantaloupe Gazpacho

Ingredients:

- 1 lb. sliced cantaloupe
- 2 tbsp. port wine
- A dusting of finely grated nutmeg
- 2 tbsp. sugar, brown, or agave

Instructions:

1. In a bowl, mix together cantaloupe, port, and sugar.
2. Let it sit in the freezer for 4 hours.
3. Place in a blender and blend.
4. Put some nutmeg dusting.
5. Serve in a cup or shotglass.

Creamy Hummus

Ingredients:

- 19 oz. canned chickpeas
- 1 cup chicken stock
- ¼ tsp. sesame oil
- 2 tbsp. olive oil
- ½ tsp. salt

Instructions:

1. In a food processor, put chickpeas, chicken stock, sesame oil, olive oil, and salt together. Grind.
2. Add chicken stock if necessary.
3. Let it cool then serve. Serve it either with oven-toasted corn chips, flatbreads, or toast points.

Watermelon and Ginger Granite

Ingredients:

- 3 cups watermelon juice
- ½ cup honey
- 1 cup water
- A pinch of ground nutmeg
- 1 whole clove
- ½ tsp. lemon zest
- 1 tsp. ginger
- 1 tsp. salt

Instructions:

1. Put together honey, water, nutmeg, clove, lemon zest, ginger, and salt in a pan. Allow them to boil.
2. Let the mixture cool then strain.
3. Put the mixture or syrup on the watermelon juice.
4. Put the juice and syrup mixture in a bowl.
5. Place in the freezer for three hours. For every 15 minutes, stir using a sauce whisk or anything that can function the same.

Quick Banana Sorbet

Ingredients:

- 3 pcs. bananas, peeled
- 2 tbsp. honey
- 1/8 tsp. ground cardamom
- 1 tbsp. grated ginger
- 3 cups ice
- ¼ tsp. salt

Instructions:

1. Blend bananas, cardamom, ginger, honey, and salt until smooth.
2. Add some ice and continue to blend. You can add more ice if necessary.
3. Serve and enjoy.

Marinated Tuna Steak

Ingredients:

- 4 slices tuna steaks
- 1/3 cup soy sauce
- 1 tbsp. cider vinegar
- 3 tbsp. olive oil
- 2 tbsp. chopped parsley
- 1 tbsp. chopped rosemary
- ½ tsp. chopped oregano
- 1/8 tsp. garlic powder

Instructions:

1. Put together olive oil, soy sauce, parsley, cider vinegar, rosemary, and oregano in a bowl. Mix well to create a marinade mixture.
2. Using a gallon plastic bag, put tuna steaks and marinade mixture. Allow the mixture to coat the tuna by turning the bag over. Leave inside the refrigerator for 30 minutes.
3. Put a small amount of oil on the grill grate. Cook tuna for about 5 minutes per side. Put some of the remaining marinade mixtures on tuna every few minutes.

Honey Roasted Potatoes

Ingredients:

- 2 lb. cubed red potatoes
- 2 tbsp. honey
- 2 tbsp. olive oil
- ½ tsp. crushed rosemary
- 1 tsp. salt
- 1 tsp. mustard powder
- Pepper, to taste

Instructions:

1. Set the oven to 375 °F.
2. Make the honey mixture by mixing honey, olive oil, salt, pepper, rosemary, and mustard powder in a small bowl.
3. Spray some nonstick spray on the baking pan.
4. Put potatoes in the pan and baste with the honey mixture. Place in the preheated oven and cook for about 35 minutes.

Kale Banana Smoothie

Ingredients:

- 16 oz. coconut water, chilled
- 1 pc. banana
- Half avocado, peeled and sliced
- ½ cup kale
- 1/8 lemon juice
- A pinch of cayenne pepper

Instructions:

1. Blend all the ingredients until smooth.
2. Put it in a glass then serve.

Maple Salmon

Ingredients:

- 1 lb. salmon
- ¼ cup maple syrup
- 2 tbsp. Dijon mustard
- 2 tbsp. soy sauce
- Parsley
- Salt and pepper, to taste

Instructions:

1. Make a syrup mixture by combining soy sauce, Dijon mustard, and maple syrup in a bowl.
2. On a baking dish, put salmon.
3. Coat it with the syrup mixture and leave it for an hour in a refrigerator. Don't forget to cover it.
4. Bake it for 20 minutes in a 400°F preheated oven.

Vegetable Broth

Ingredients:

- 1 tbsp. oil
- 2 leeks, sliced
- 2 carrots, sliced
- 2 ribs celery
- ¼ tsp. salt
- 8 cups water

To make the soup:

- 1 tbsp. oil
- 2 cups potatoes, diced
- 1 cup mushrooms, diced
- 1.5 cups cauliflower, diced
- 1 cup onion, diced
- 1 cup celery, diced
- 1 cup carrot, diced
- 1.5 cups red beans, cooked
- 2 sprigs rosemary
- 4 sprigs thyme
- 2 cups spinach

Instructions:

1. To a pot on medium heat, add oil and leeks.
2. Cook for about three minutes or until they start to soften up.

3. Add carrots and top of a few celery stalks with leaves.
4. Cover with water.
5. Add salt. Bring to a simmer and cook until carrots are very tender but not mushy.
6. Turn off the heat and let it cool down a little.
7. When the broth has cooled down, strain out the veggies.
8. Remove carrots and set aside.
9. Squeeze most of the liquid out of the leeks and celery.

To cook the soup:

1. Add carrots to some of the broth and blend.
2. With a pot on medium heat, add oil, onions, raw carrots, and celery. Cook until onions are translucent, approximately 3 to 5 minutes.
3. Add broth, potatoes, and herbs.
4. Bring to a simmer and cook for ten minutes.
5. Add cauliflower and red beans.
6. Simmer for another five minutes.
7. Add the package of frozen green beans and cook until the potatoes and cauliflower are tender, approximately for another five minutes.
8. At the end of cooking, add two cups of spinach.

Spinach and Chickpeas

Ingredients:

- 3 tbsp. extra virgin olive oil
- 1 large onion, thinly sliced
- 4 cloves garlic, minced
- 1 tbsp. grated ginger
- ½ container grape tomatoes
- 1 tsp. crushed red pepper flakes
- 1 large can of chickpeas
- Sea salt, to taste

Instructions:

1. Add extra virgin olive oil to a large skillet.
2. Add onion and cook until onion starts to brown.
3. Add garlic, ginger, tomatoes, and red pepper flakes.
4. Cook for about 3 to 4 minutes.
5. Serve and enjoy.

Apple Cinnamon Smash Oatmeal

Ingredients:

- 1 ½ cups plain almond milk
- 1 cup oats
- 1 large Granny Smith apple
- ¼ tsp. ground cinnamon
- 2 tbsp. toasted walnut pieces

Instructions:

1. Heat apple and oats together in low to medium fire for about 5 minutes.
2. Add cinnamon.
3. Serve hot.

Fruit and Dark Greens Salad

Ingredients:

- For the Salad:
- 1 cup watermelon
- 1 cup cucumber, sliced or spiral
- ½ cup raspberries
- 1 sliced avocado
- 1 cup baby broccoli
- 1 cup papaya
- ½ cup toasted almonds
- 4 cups baby kale

For the dressing:

- ½ cup olive oil
- ½ cup master tonic
- ¼ cup goji berries
- 4 dates
- A pinch of sea salt

For the tonic:

- ¼ cup garlic, minced
- ¼ cup onion, chopped
- 2 tbsp. horseradish, minced
- 2 knobs of turmeric, chopped
- 1 jalapeno pepper, chopped
- 32 oz. organic apple cider vinegar

- ¼ cup fresh ginger, chopped
- 1 fresh lemon juice

Instructions:
1. To make the salad:
2. Mix all ingredients except almonds.
3. Toss well.

To make the dressing:
1. Mix master tonic, olive oil, and salt.
2. Add dates and goji berries to a blender. Blend until smooth.
3. Drizzle dressing on the salad and sprinkle toasted almonds.

To make the master tonic:
1. Add all ingredients to apple cider vinegar.
2. Blend all ingredients just until they are mixed.
3. Let tonic sit in a jar for 1 to 2 weeks, shaking periodically.
4. Strain the ingredients and add the remaining vinegar mixture into a jar with a top.

Spinach, Feta, and Tomato Omelet

Ingredients:

- Cooking spray
- ¼ cup Roma tomatoes, chopped
- ¾ cup Egg Beaters Liquid Egg Whites
- 2 tbsp. fat-reduced feta cheese, crumbled
- 1/8 tsp. ground black pepper
- ¼ cup baby spinach leaves, chopped

Instructions:

1. Spray small amounts of cooking spray in a nonstick skillet. Heat over medium heat.
2. Cook the Egg Beaters in the skillet, and season with pepper. Cook for 2 minutes.
3. Lift the edges to cook the other side of the egg. Cook for 3 more minutes.
4. Top half of the omelet with tomatoes, spinach, and feta cheese. Fold the other half of the omelet over the filling.
5. Serve.

Salmon and Asparagus

Ingredients:

- 2 salmon fillets, around 5 oz. each
- 14 oz. young potatoes
- 8 asparagus spears, trimmed and halved
- 2 handfuls cherry tomatoes
- 1 handful basil leaves
- 2 tbsp. extra-virgin olive oil
- 1 tbsp. balsamic vinegar

Instructions:

1. Heat oven to 428°F.
2. Arrange potatoes on a baking dish.
3. Drizzle potatoes with 1 tbsp. extra-virgin olive oil.
4. Roast potatoes for 20 minutes, or until golden brown.
5. Place asparagus into the baking dish together with potatoes.
6. Roast in the oven for another 15 minutes.
7. Arrange cherry tomatoes and salmon among the vegetables.
8. Drizzle with balsamic vinegar and the remaining olive oil.
9. Roast for 10 to 15 minutes, or until salmon is cooked.
10. Throw in a handful of basil leaves before transferring everything to a serving dish.
11. Serve while hot.

Grilled Eggplant

Ingredients:

- 2 small eggplants or 1 large eggplant, around 1¼ to 1½ lbs. in total, sliced into ½-inch thick rounds
- 2 tbsp. extra-virgin olive oil
- A pinch of salt

Instructions:

1. Preheat the grill using the medium-high setting.
2. Toss eggplant slices and olive oil in a bowl.
3. Sprinkle it with salt to taste.
4. Toss ingredients again.
5. Place eggplant slices into the grill.
6. Turn over to the other side after about 4 minutes, or until charred spots have appeared on the underside.
7. Continue grilling until eggplant slices have become tender.
8. When storing, place it into an airtight container once it has cooled down, and then refrigerate. Grilled eggplant can last for up to 4 days in a chilled condition.

Physical Activity and Heartburn Management

Beyond diet, there could potentially be a way to manage heartburn symptoms. For many people, physical activity is not merely about staying fit or losing weight. It can serve a crucial role in managing various health conditions, including heartburn. Research suggests that moderate-intensity exercise can help decrease symptoms of GERD (Gastroesophageal Reflux Disease), a severe form of heartburn.

Understanding the Connection

The connection between exercise and heartburn is not as straightforward as it might seem. On the one hand, regular, moderate exercise can help reduce the symptoms of heartburn by stimulating digestion and promoting a healthy weight. Carrying excess weight, particularly around the abdomen, puts additional pressure on your stomach and can exacerbate heartburn symptoms.

On the other hand, high-intensity exercises or workouts that involve a lot of jarring or bending over can trigger heartburn.

Movements like these can cause the lower esophageal sphincter, a muscle that acts as a one-way valve between the esophagus and stomach, to relax, allowing acid to flow back up into the esophagus.

Choosing the Right Exercise

Given this complex relationship between exercise and heartburn, it's essential to choose the right type of workout. Low-impact exercises such as walking, cycling, or swimming are typically safe options for people with heartburn. Yoga and gentle stretching exercises can also be beneficial, but be cautious of poses that involve bending over or lying flat on your back for extended periods.

It's recommended to wait at least two hours after eating before exercising, as this gives your body time to digest your food. If you exercise too soon after eating, you may experience heartburn or acid reflux.

Hydration and Heartburn

Staying well-hydrated during exercise is crucial for everyone, but it's particularly important for people with heartburn. Drinking plenty of water can help dilute stomach acid and reduce the risk of heartburn. However, be careful not to overdo it, as too much water can lead to bloating, which can worsen heartburn symptoms.

Heartburn-Friendly Workout Plan

A sample heartburn-friendly workout plan might include a gentle warm-up routine, followed by 20-30 minutes of low-impact aerobic exercise, such as walking or cycling. After this, you might do some light strength training exercises, ensuring to avoid any movements that strain your abdominal muscles overly. Finish your workout with a cool-down routine that includes gentle stretches.

Remember, every person is unique, so what works for one person might not work for another. Listen to your body and adjust your workout plan as necessary. If you're not sure where to start, consider consulting with a healthcare professional or a fitness specialist.

Physical activity is an essential part of a heartburn management strategy. But like everything else, it needs to be balanced and tailored to your specific needs. Always remember to consult your healthcare provider before starting any new fitness regimen.

Other Lifestyle Remedies to Manage Heartburn

Aside from diet and exercise, there are several other lifestyle interventions you can implement to manage heartburn effectively. These remedies complement your dietary and physical activity efforts to create a comprehensive heartburn management plan.

Stress Management

Stress can significantly exacerbate heartburn symptoms, making stress management strategies a crucial part of any heartburn management plan. Techniques might include mindfulness exercises, deep-breathing techniques, yoga, and adequate sleep. Reducing your stress levels can have a calming effect on your entire body, including your digestive system.

Weight Management

Maintaining a healthy weight can also help manage heartburn. Excess weight can put pressure on your abdomen, pushing up your stomach and causing acid to back up into your esophagus. Therefore, if you're overweight, losing even a few pounds can help relieve your heartburn symptoms.

Smoking and Alcohol

Both smoking and alcohol can contribute to heartburn. Smoking weakens the lower esophageal sphincter, the muscle that keeps stomach acid from backing up into the esophagus, while alcohol can increase the production of stomach acid. If you smoke or drink alcohol regularly, consider cutting back or quitting to help manage heartburn symptoms.

Clothing Choices

Tight clothing, particularly around your waist, can put pressure on your abdomen and the lower esophageal sphincter, leading to heartburn. Opt for loose-fitting clothing to minimize this risk.

Proper Posture

Practicing good posture can also help prevent heartburn by reducing abdominal pressure. Try to keep your body upright, especially during and after meals.

Adequate Sleep

Getting enough sleep is another essential lifestyle remedy for heartburn. Lack of sleep can exacerbate stress and heartburn symptoms. Moreover, your sleeping position can affect heartburn symptoms - it's best to keep your head elevated to prevent stomach acid from flowing back into the esophagus.

Medication Review

Certain medications, including some pain relievers and antihistamines, can cause heartburn. If you suspect your medication might be contributing to your heartburn, consult a healthcare professional. Never stop taking prescribed medication without first consulting your healthcare provider.

Remember, while these lifestyle remedies can significantly aid in managing heartburn, they are not a complete solution. It's important to consult with a healthcare provider to create a comprehensive, personalized heartburn management plan. Implementing these strategies in combination with dietary and physical activity changes can lead to a significant improvement in heartburn symptoms, enhancing your overall quality of life.

A Two-Week Guide to Managing Heartburn

Now that you've acquired knowledge on managing heartburn through diet, exercise, and other lifestyle remedies, let's summarize how to implement this in a two-week plan.

Day 1-3: Dietary Changes

Identify and eliminate heartburn-triggering foods (spicy foods, citrus fruits, high-fat foods).

Start a food diary to track your meals and heartburn episodes.

Day 4-5: Meal Planning

Opt for smaller, frequent meals instead of three large ones.

Avoid eating 2-3 hours before bedtime for better digestion.

Day 6-7: Exercise Incorporation

Introduce light exercises like walking or yoga.

Avoid exercising immediately after meals to minimize heartburn symptoms.

Day 8-10: Wardrobe Adjustment

Review your wardrobe and wear loose-fitting clothes, especially around the waist.

Tight clothing can increase abdominal pressure, leading to heartburn.

Day 11-12: Posture and Sleep Adjustment

Maintain good posture during and after meals.

Elevate your head while sleeping to prevent acid reflux.

Day 13-14: Medication Review

Consult a healthcare professional and review your medications.

Some antihistamines and pain relievers can contribute to heartburn.

Never stop taking prescribed medication without medical advice.

Remember, everyone is different, so adjust these strategies as needed. Track your progress and consult with a healthcare provider to create a comprehensive heartburn management plan. This two-week guide can be a starting point for long-term changes to manage heartburn and improve your overall quality of life.

Conclusion

The heartburn relief diet plan is designed to provide comprehensive guidance on managing acid reflux through dietary choices. It not only advises on what foods to consume and avoid but also emphasizes the significance of portion control, as excessive meal consumption often triggers acid reflux symptoms.

In order to effectively follow the heartburn relief diet plan, it is crucial to maintain discipline and adhere to the recommended meal plans. Additionally, documenting your journey can prove beneficial in identifying specific foods that may exacerbate your symptoms, enabling you to make informed adjustments.

However, it is essential to remember that seeking professional medical advice before embarking on any diet plan is of utmost importance. Consulting a healthcare professional will ensure that the heartburn relief diet plan aligns with your individual needs and medical condition, promoting your overall well-being.

www.ingramcontent.com/pod-product-compliance
Lightning Source LLC
LaVergne TN
LVHW012037060526
838201LV00061B/4655